You Are Not Getting Older, You Are Getting Better

CHRISTINA WALDMAN

authorHOUSE®

AuthorHouse™
1663 Liberty Drive
Bloomington, IN 47403
www.authorhouse.com
Phone: 1-800-839-8640

First published by AuthorHouse 4/9/2010

ISBN: 978-1-4490-9908-4 (sc)
ISBN: 978-1-4490-9909-1 (e)

*Printed in the United States of America
Bloomington, Indiana*

This book is printed on acid-free paper.

I dedicate this book to God for giving me so many talents. He put writing into my life, giving me inspiration to be able to communicate with people and to let them know how beautiful and important they all are.

HELLO, WOMEN FROM ALL OVER the world! I love each one of you, and this book is just for you.

Think of this as your beauty bible – your best friend! It should be on your night table, and you should carry it in your bag and read as many times as you feel you need it.

It is a very easy and fun book to read, and I know it will help all of you.

I will also give you some recipes, and exercises that will be very helpful.

XO

Chapter One

ABOUT ME

I was a makeup-artist for nine years, at a midtown department store. Today I freelance for a number of well-known companies. Due to my everyday contact with women from all over the world, women of all ages, I decided to write this book. Their main concern is the same: "I am getting old!" Well, remember something. Age is only a number. Now of course, as we mature the skin texture of a fifty-year-old it is not the same as a 20-year-old, but there are many things you can do to have a great skin.

Mind and body go together. Much has to do with the way you were brought up, your friends, your insecurities, fears, self esteem, satisfaction with what you look like – *Oh, I wish I was taller, I wish I was thinner, I wish I wish I wish!*

Stop right there! It's fine to admire people that are different than you, but never wish to be someone else other than your self! You are beautiful just the way you are. Could you imagine if we all looked alike? Be happy with yourself, love yourself the way you are, and you will be much happier.

Sometimes we see a very fat woman with a gorgeous guy, and we say to ourselves, *what does he see in her?* Well, you know what? This girl has so much confidence in herself that the guy can't even see her not-so-pleasant figure. Of course, I do not agree that a woman should her self go - I don't care what the problem is, you should always take care of yourself, for yourself.

You can make yourself look very ugly; however, you can also make yourself look very beautiful. Attitude is very important. Usually when a person is insecure, she talks loudly about material things, and worries about how a man might like her to look. That's another big no-no! You should be yourself. The guy is going to love you for what you are, so try to love the way that you look. You will see great results. What I am trying to say to you is that everything comes from the inside of you, and immediately will show on the outside. Every morning, before you get out of bed, say "Thank you God, for my life and my health, for who I am, and for one more day of victory." It will make you feel great! Go to the bathroom; look at yourself in the mirror, and say: "I love you just the way you are! You are beautiful and I love you. Everything is working the way you want. You are young, beautiful, and healthy. I love everyone, I am loved by everyone!" Believe me, it works!

I don't care if it makes you late for work – do it every day! The mirror is like magic. Seeing yourself, and talking to yourself, will make the words come true!

XO

Chapter Two

AGE 20 - 27

What a beautiful age! But it is so complicated: changes, big changes. Before, you lived with your parents. Now you have your own place, expenses, and the freedom to as you please. Sometimes you feel homesick. But at the same time, your own place comes first.

You have a job which you give your best to grow, and at the same time you are becoming independent, as far as money is concerned.

You have new friends, and you hang out in different places, drinking, smoking, and spending money on expensive clothes. Labels are very important to you. Don't make the mistake of going on a date, and, after dinner, when the bill comes, offering to split the bill.

I am not being old fashioned. If you out with a guy who you think could be your future husband, don't do it. This is one of the big mistakes that girls make. Today, man and woman are equal in many ways, but the husband should always be the "bus driver" of the house. I am always in favor of a woman pursuing a career, but things get to the point where a couple, instead of working out their problems, gets a divorce instead. It is very sad the way things are going.

Of course, when you are married and you both work, it is natural to share bills. After all, you are growing together.

Now, listen, you are too young to get married. These are just examples and advice for the future. Ok?

Most important, take it easy on the drinking, smoking, and tanning. They will all make you age before time, and you will look 10 years older by the time you are 40. They are poison for the skin, and very few people get away with it.

As far as implants, don't do it before you 35, unless they are absolutely necessary. Let your natural beauty flow!

Very important: don't jump into bed with just any guy. Have self-respect! That is the only way you will be loved and respected. Don't be too available, especially if you really like the guy. Go slow. go slow, take your time, let him come after you. And when you sure he is serious about you, you can let your feelings go.

I spoke to our floor director while I was working in a midtown department store. He's a nice looking guy in his late twenties. I asked him: "What kind of a girl do you want for your wife??

His answer was great. "I want a wife, a friend, and a good mother for my children. I want her to be close with my parents, because my family is very important to me." His parents are Italian, of course. He also mentioned that he wanted what every man wants, but girls make that so easy that guys have no chance to pursue the one he really wants.

Now, let's get to your looks!

Use and abuse eye make-up. Do your hair anyway you like. That's the age where everything looks good - so of course, use your good taste. Go slow on face make-up. Use bronzers, shimmers, and smoky eyes, of course, matching your eye color and hair.

I just want you to know that everything I say it's because I met many girls your age that made so many mistakes, and today, they are so unhappy. I don't want the same thing to happen to you. That's part of beauty too.

Xoxoxoxo!

Chapter Three

AGES 27 – 30

Unless you have great self esteem, and you feel secure about who you are, this age is very difficult for most girls.

If you don't feel secure, this age could be the beginning of the feeling that you are getting old, and you need to get married as soon as possible. You are going to start to find wrinkles that do not exist. You see, your mind commands your body and soul, so that every negative thought you have will come back to you. Every positive thing you say and think will come back to you. So remember these words! They are very precious.

Some girls have the attitude that they think they are better and more beautiful than others. This is wrong! If your parents brought you up saying that you are the best, its fine; but if they tell say you are better and more beautiful than others, that's definitely wrong. Because when you grow up and encounter the outside world, you will find out that things are very different. Then your problems will start.

Perhaps you will choose a guy that will be easy for you to manipulate - deep down inside, however, he's not the man you want for your husband. You might always look for friends that you are able to manipulate, or friends just like you - but you will become a "plastic woman," and inside you may be beautiful, sweet and loving, but you will always be afraid to let it go. Be your own self! Then you will find true happiness.

Now, the 27 to 30 year old girls.

Skin:

Very natural, very light makeup. Use tinted moisturizer with SPF. There is oil-free and regular. If you have skin problem where you need more coverage, you can use a liquid foundation. Make sure you apply with a brush – it's important to have an even look. Don't use foundation powder, because that will make you look older. After that, use a good mineral powder or bronzer to give you a natural glow. Then use a natural color blush.

Just a little touch! Don't forget: always use a primer under your tinted moisturizer or foundation. Not only will your pores will be protected, but it will help to reduce redness, especially for girls with red spots. It will also keep your makeup on for about 10 hours.

Eyes:

Please don't forget your eyebrows. They are the frame of your eyes, and should always be well-shaped.

Eyes are the expression of the face. Your eyes express happiness, sadness, worry, and so many other emotions. So always have the perfect colors: blue eyes, no blue shadow; green eyes, no green shadow; brown and hazel eyes, any color will go.

Daytime:

A neutral bone color all over the eyes, use a medium-size soft brush, and apply gently, on the crease, a brown, dark plum, or a mixture of grey, blue, purple, all in one. Laura Mercier has a color called Twilight Grey; it goes with every eye color. After application, use a blending brush to make sure the eye color is even. Some eyeliner and mascara, and you are all done to start your day! You must look your best every single day.

Nighttime:

Make the eye crease darker; darken your eye corner, bringing up your eyes towards the end of your brows. Always use a blending brush. Brushes are your most important tools to get perfect eye makeup; afterwards, wet the tip of your brush and deep on the darker eye shadow, and do your bottom line, a little neutral shimmer under the brow bone, and the inside corner of the eye. I will have a picture at the end of the book. A shimmer all over the face - always make sure the color of your face makeup, matches your neck.

If you can't afford expensive makeup, try Neutrogena or L'oreal Cover Girl.

Everything I said about you will help you. Believe me, there's more in life than just a beautiful face.

Remember: dress for you, look beautiful for you! When you look in the mirror and like the way you look, everyone will look at you with the same eyes. And always be the Real You - I am sure you will find your other half soon.

Xoxoxoxoxo!

Chapter Four

Age 30

Congratulations! You have become a woman. Someone with lots of experience told me when a woman turns 30, she loses her baby face, gains a brighter look, and becomes a woman. It's true! My taste for men changed, I looked prettier, I felt sexier, and so much more secure of myself. There wasn't a moment when I thought I was growing old. I thought I was getting better.

In Brazil, they made a song for a woman of thirty, and I remember it until this day. But it took me a while to understand the real meaning of the words.

For some girls, turning is not a great thing, especially if they don't have a steady boy friend. That's their main concern. Of course I am not saying all of you, but about eighty percent of all girls.

Suddenly their girlfriends are getting married, and they feel that they must make new single friends who feel the same way they do. Don't worry; what's yours is on the way! But if you get anxious, you will block that person's entrance into your life. There is a right time and place for everything.

Before you go to sleep, thank God for the day you've had, even if wasn't the best. Thank God for your health and your job. After that close your eyes, take a deep breath, and exhale. Do this five times, without thinking about anything.

Good, you feel relaxed! Now, with your eyes closed, see yourself with the guy of your dreams. You are both happy, holding hands. Imagine a place, and the clothes you are both wearing, and say to yourself in silence: I am so happy I finally met my husband-to-be. He is just the way I wanted, and we love each other the way we are. He proposed to me, and soon we will be married. We are perfect for each other. Thank you!

Do it every night, before you go to sleep. During the day, when you are alone, close your eyes for a few seconds. You will see yourself with him again.

I guarantee you this works! When you think or say something, you attract thoughts and words to you, so make sure not to say or think negative things.

Sometimes, I hear girls say: "Today is not my day. My hair looks terrible. I don't like what I am wearing. I hate my job. Everything is going wrong in my life."

When I hear this, I tell them: "Erase all the words you just said, and say just the opposite. You have to learn to watch every single word that comes out of your mouth, because it will come back to you. Our minds are very powerful, so please be careful with your words and thoughts. "When a bad thought comes, sing, or call a friend to talk about good things, until you able to control that part of your mind. We all have our days, but try to make the best out of it."

When many of my regulars come to have their makeup done, they say: "Christina, you always make me feel good!" But you must learn to follow what I say. I went through many things in my life, and believe me if I didn't love my self the way I do, I would not be writing this book today. I love you all so very much that even though I don't know you personally, I want the best for you. I will try to help you in every way I can, but *please* listen to me and go with the flow. It is very important to have friends that you can learn from, so that you are happy most the time. A good friend should have a head on her shoulders. Someone who won't let you talk about negative things.

I always try to be positive. I am happy most of the time, and I am always hoping for better things to come. I am always grateful for everything. Don't think I don't have my bad days! I simply learned how to have control of my emotions.

But back to you!

Make-up should be very natural skin make-up, with tinted moisturizer, followed by a mineral powder softly applied. This will give you a beautiful glow. Eyes need to be a light color all over, with lots of eye liner and mascara. Don't forget the eyebrows! Wait for thin eyebrows – those will only look good when you are in your late seventies.

Of course, the look I just gave you is a daytime look. When you are out at night, you need drama on your eyes. Apply a dark crease, with dark on the outside corner. You can also go all smoky. It's up to you!

If you need a lot of coverage, and have a little acne, you should use foundation and translucent powder. Apply the powder very softly with a powder brush. No mineral powder or shimmer at all. Use a little bronzer, use a little blush, and line your lips all over with a natural color gloss. I am sure you will look beautiful.

Hair must always cover the neck. Even if you don't like long hair, you should at least have it long enough to cover your neck. It's very feminine. Short hair is not for everybody. After a while, it becomes boring.

Xoxoxoxoxoxoxoxo!

XO

Chapter Five

Ages 35 to 39

Now girls, I want you to pay attention to everything I have to say. It's really very important. I feel like I am everyone's mother. It is great! I have two sons, but no girls. But today, after being in contact with all of you, I wish I had a daughter too. But now you are all my daughters, and I want to see you happy and satisfied with your lives.

Let's get back to business. I want you to know that when you turn 35, your hormones start to change. This happens to every one of us. You must go to your doctor. Make sure to start taking calcium. Exercise is also a must.

Most of us, when we turn 35, we start to loose collagen little by little. Collagen keeps our skin firm. We are able to keep the collage in our bodies by taking natural vitamins, eating the right food, and exercising. I will give a little recipe at the end.

Today there are so many things we can do to look younger without looking ridiculous. This is a critical age for almost everyone. Girls get so involved with their careers that they forget to be more feminine.

In order to have a partner at this point, you have to forget work when you are together. You should be together as man and woman, not as business people. I have seen many cases like that and at the end, the relationship is over. Men like women to have their own personalities: soft, loving, intelligent. A wife should be a friend. After all, after a few years of marriage, you end up being best friends. It is a different type of love.

I want you to know that some of us were meant to get married and have a family, and some of us were meant to be single.

I will be talking about your personal life a little more, before I get to the makeup and hair part. I want you to listen to what I have to say. It will help you a great deal.

Last week a friend of mine called me to invite me to her birthday party. I laughed and said: "Finally you turned 21!"

She said, "I wish it was true."

"How old are you going to be?" I asked.

"Thirty-seven, but I told everyone 32. Please keep it to yourself."

She is so concerned with age. She has already done everything to have a perfect body, and she has done many things to have a perfect face. She looks 35, or at most 37.

She is afraid to get old. She dresses like a twenty-year-old girl, and it looks terrible. I would never say anything though, because she won't listen.

I have another friend who is going to be forty. Her boyfriend is 22 years old. Yes, 22! She looks 35, but if you see them together, you can tell the difference in age right away. We were talking, and she told me that she was very depressed, because he told her it was time to end the relationship. They were together since he was 20.

"He said that when he felt that he wanted to be free from our relationship, he would tell me. He hoped I would do the same. Unfortunately he told me first."

I said: "You brought this onto yourself. We are our own worst enemies, and you just didn't listen.

He is right. He wants to be free and enjoy his single life. Now you are gorgeous and intelligent. You have a fantastic job. You should just be happy for the two years you spent together! You have to be open to meet Mr. Right. I know what you are going through, but don't think you lost. You knew from the beginning that this would happen.

Now after few months, she is almost over him. She is always calling to find out how she is. She finally asked him not to call anymore, because she was trying very hard to get him out of her life.

Almost a year later, she met a doctor at a friend's party, and they are getting alone fine. He is 43 and was never married. He told her that after he met her, he thinks it is finally the right time. They both agreed not to have children, and she is happy! I met him last year when I went to Brazil on vacation. He is a great guy, and I am sure its going to work out for them.

I personally think if the man is six years younger than you, and looks older than you it is okay. But no more than that! Believe me it doesn't work. You might say: "My friend has been married for years, and he is fifteen years younger than his wife." Well, sometimes it works, because her self-esteem is sky-high. She probably takes good care of herself. But in most cases it does not work.

Love yourself, believe in your potential, take care of your inner beauty, and of course your body, face and soul. If you do this you won't have a problem. Men know when women are needy. If you come off this way, you will lose.

Enjoy this beautiful age! You are growing to be even more beautiful than you already are.

Beauty:

Day cream moisturizer with SPF eye cream. Don't forget to warm up the cream in your hands! Press it against your skin, so it gets right into the pores. Do the same with eye cream and night eye cream. And no night cream, unless you really need it. At the end of the book, I will teach you how to do your own facial at home.

After the cream, some foundation primer and foundation mixed with tinted moisturizer will make you look young and fresh, and will give you great coverage. Don't forget your eyebrows: very little powder or light blush, applied with a fluffy brush. Eyes should be your natural color for the day, with eye liner applied very softly. Use lots of mascara, and curl your lashes. Light lips are important, too.

At night, everything goes on the eyes. Don't forget smoky eyes, light lips, thin lips and light color lipstick.

If you have long hair, try to have it with soft waves. This makes you look younger. Keep it shoulder-length and straight, with a part between the middle and the side and some volume at the ends. No flat irons please!

I am sure you are looking goooood, young, classy, and sexy.

Enjoy yourself, and easy on the wine and cigarettes.

Xoxoxoxoxoxoxoxoxo!

Chapter Six

AGE 40

Wow!!!!!! Happy happy happy birthday, feliz aniversario! You finally hit the glorious forty. Congratulations!

When I turned 40, I had a fantastic birthday party. People thought I was 28. Hard to believe? Yes, but it is very very true. Not only didn't I look my age, but I felt as if I was 20. I didn't act twenty, but I felt twenty.

When you turn 40, you become a totally new person. You feel beautiful and sexy. Your sex life increases, too. My husband used to say that he wished I was 40 every day! Not that I was cold before, but I became full of life, and I loved myself even more. It was such a great feeling. In our minds, we might not feel that we are not so young, but not old either. We are somewhere on the border.

Somehow, there is such a desire to look good and change our looks for better. It is true when I say that we become like a lioness, as far as our sex lives are concerned.

Forty to fifty are the most important and glorious years of our lives. And yet, that's when men experience their own menopause. They change in every way. It takes a long time for them to accept that they are 40. They start to get nervous with their first gray or loss of hair. It is unbelievable but true! Of course, not all men are like that, but maybe 80% are.

On the other hand, we women have control of our situations. We change our hair color, style, makeup, way of dressing, and fix those fine lines that begin to show in the face (no Botox please!). If we need to fix our boobs, it's fine. See how many advantages we have over men? Going to the gym is a must, especially for the arms, legs and tummy. Let's make everything hard!

There are gyms for everyone. If you cannot afford a famous one, there are others for you. This country is so blessed, that there are no excuses for you not to take care of your face and body. Never forget you inner beauty, it is very important.

They say that Brazilian women are beautiful and their bodies are perfect because of plastic surgery. This is false! Yes they might have a breast lift if needed or a few applications on the face. These are so natural that you can't even tell. Maybe laser peeling, which is good, and does not cause harm. Very little breast implants, because Brazilian men, like all Latin men, don't care about big breasts. They like a beautiful ass, pardon my French.

But most importantly, Brazilian women go to the gym almost every day. They love their bodies, like we all do. But the body must be taken care of, no matter if you are rich or poor.

If you are overweight, you probably have a beautiful face, like most overweight women. So please, put a picture of a woman with a beautiful body on your refrigerator door, so you will think twice before you eat. Love yourself and your body. Feel beautiful and discipline yourself. Close your eyes and imagine the way you would like to look. Say to yourself: "I am happy, because I lost all the weight I needed. Now my body is perfect. I am in charge of my body, and I eat enough to just keep myself in shape." You know you are your own best friend, not your worst enemy. And don't forget plenty of exercise for you, so as you lose weight your muscles become firm.

If you are married, you should take better care of yourself. Being married when you are forty is very important. If you have a husband at home, you don't want him looking at other women and desiring other women because you look like a rag. Don't think that because you are married and have children you have a secure marriage. That's when you really should look your best. Most importantly, drink lots of water. Water is good for everything: health, body, and your beautiful face.

Most women, when become 40, start to make new decisions for their lives. This is very interesting. Do you know why?

You become mature, and wise, and really start to see that life is not all about partying. I have a very good friend who recently turned 30. She was madly in love with a 45 year old man. From the beginning, he told her that he was married, and he would not leave his wife, even though they had no children. She married him when he had nothing.

Then he became a very wealthy and well-known lawyer. She always stood by him. But my friend and the lawyer traveled together, and they went out every night. They worked together at the same law firm, so they would see each other all day, and for few hours with her on weekends, but no holidays. The affair went on for 10 years. I remember telling her: "You are throwing your best years away! You have no children and no husband!"

"I don't want children," was her answer.

When she turned 40, they went away for a long weekend. He gave her a beautiful car, and everything was fine. On Tuesday she called me around ten in the morning, and asked me if I wanted to meet her for lunch. We lived in the same building, so we met around 1:00. She looked beautiful as always, and I asked her. "What time you have to go back to the office?"

"I don't."

"You took the day off?"

"I took a permanent vacation."

I stopped and looked at her. She told me that she put an end to her 10-year affair. She was not sorry, because she was happy for ten years. She also made a deal at work, as though she was fired, and she got a great severance package. I was in shock! She was very calm, and said, "I think I want to take a long vacation. When I come back, I will think about my future."

She went to Hawaii for two months. When she came back, she started to go out, and one day she met a guy. Long story short: today she is married with no children, but very happy.

What I am trying to say is that when we turn 40, we start to see life from a different angle. Some people make the right decisions for themselves, and some people just go with the flow until one day they wake up. My advice: don't get involved with a married man. Not only will you end up hurt, but the man's wife will be hurt also. You can't ever be happy making someone else miserable. My friend was one of the lucky ones. In my next book "Let's find your other half," we are going to have lots of fun.

Now let's go back to you.

Make-up: face cream, eye cream, foundation primer, light foundation, mineral powder, and soft color blush. Eye primer, with pale rose shadow all over, and dark plum in the corner of the eyes to bring them all the way up. No crease, a little neutral shimmer shadow in the inside corner to open the eye. Use the same shadow under the brow bone very softly, and softly apply eyeliner on the bottom, with lots of mascara. Don't forget the eyebrows! At night, have dark eyes, but the rest should remain the same. Light lips, waved hair if long, and full if shoulder-length. Dress sexy, but never trashy. I am sure you all look beautiful. I will give some more tips at the end.

Xoxoxoxoxoxoxo!

XO

Chapter Seven

AGE 50

Wow Wow Wow! You just turned fifty years old. For many this is very depressing. For others means nothing, because they looked 50 when they were 40.

In the big cities, women care much more about their looks than women from other places, where they lead a simple life. They dedicate their lives to their children, home, and husband. If they have time left, they might look in the mirror.

I remember one summer; a woman on her early fifties was walking around my counter. She had five children, all teenagers, and all girls. You

Christina Waldman

could see that she had pretty features, but they looked tired. She just let herself go completely. Her roots were grayish, and her hair was a dirty-looking blonde color. She really didn't care. She was walking around with a smile on her face and she had a nice body. Her girls were gorgeous; it was their first time in New York, so for them everything was beautiful. In the morning they went to see the NBC morning show at Rockefeller Plaza, and now there she was, looking at me at the makeup display. I noticed right away that she would love to have her makeup done.

I said to myself: "You know what? I am going to do a real makeover." I asked her if she wanted to have her makeup done, and she agreed right away.

"Go mama go mama!" Her daughters said.

Those girls were so adorable, with their southern accents! I told them where to go to see things suitable for their ages, so I would be able to work on their mother without pressure.

Long story short, after I finished her makeup, I took a brush with eye shadow and covered her grey hair on the most important parts. A woman should never walk around like that, because there are many inexpensive hair colors that you can use in your own home to fix your hair.

We became friends. She told me about her life, and how she let herself go thinking only about her family, and forgetting about herself. She also told me that her husband was always looking at other woman!

I told her: "If I were him I would do the same thing. I am sure that he loves you, but he is giving you a message. I like to look at beautiful woman because my wife doesn't take care of her self."

She had a nice body, and she showed me her pictures when she was in her early twenties. Stunning beauty.

I didn't let her look in the mirror till I was done. I took her over to a full sized mirror by the counter, and told her to look at her self.

She looked at herself, and then she looked at me. She said: "I don't believe that's me! And my hair too?" Then she hugged me.

"No crying!" I said. "Watch your makeup."

The kids came back, and when they saw their mother, they told her she looked like a movie star! Then they kissed her. She looked stunning! Even my co-workers told me after she left: "Christina, she looks fantastic."

All she bought was lipstick, because she didn't have the money to spend on expensive makeup. So I made a list of what she should buy in a drugstore. I felt so good, because I made somebody happy.

She really looked beautiful, and that gives me joy. She was only 41 years old.

What I am trying to say is that even if a woman doesn't take care of herself, deep down inside, they all like to look beautiful. Money is not the issue because they can find what they need in a drugstore. It might not be the best quality, but at least you can make yourself look beautiful, and improve yourself. Just make sure you get the right color foundation: check that it is not too thick, check your neck when choosing the color, and most importantly check your skin to see if it is oily, dry, or mixed. Of course, choose the right color eyeshadow – make sure it matches your hair and eye color. Match the lipstick with your eye shadow and your clothes. Pink lipstick is a no-no with an orange top. It matters a lot when you do the right matching. Today it is not necessary to match handbags and shoes, but your face and hair are totally different.

Now let's get into the facts. When we turn fifty, it is a tragedy, a big tragedy. Especially during the summer, when you see all the girls walking around in shorts, mini skirts, mini blouses showing their flat and hard tummies. Of course, they're in their twenties. You look and think, "What happened to me? I can't dress like that anymore." Men just love looking at them. It is a big shock for most women.

They think they already lived half a century, and there is no turning back. Some women go into depression, especially if they were never married and have no children. Other women try to look and dress like their daughters. Menopause starts changing the body. It is a real mess.

You have to realize that you are not just getting older, but you are getting better. Sure, that is easy for me to say, but you're not in my shoes. Believe me, I know how you feel.

But don't get desperate! It only make things worse. I've seen cases where the husband left his wife for a much younger girl. Poor him, he is such a loser. You a winner so don't feel bad, not even for a minute. These types of men are so insecure; they need to prove to themselves that they still got it. I really do feel sorry for a man that marries a child. It is like marrying his own daughter, and sooner or later, the girl will start going out with a man closer to her age.

So why should you be depressed and let yourself go? You are much stronger than he is. Pick yourself up, get in shape, and fight that fear of growing old. You are not old.

Remember that fear, doubt and anger are not parts of your life. I know it is not easy going through menopause. I was lucky: when I had my last period, I went to the doctor, and he told me that was it. I went home and I cried so much. I was only 47, and I was crying because I realized that I could no longer be a mother.

My younger son Joshua was 23 years old, and he was living with me at the time. When he got home from work he saw me in bed. He asked me if I was sick. I started crying again and when I told him what had happened, he started laughing, and told me "Mom, you are a grandmother! How can you think about having babies?"

I told him that it was the idea of being unable to have babies, because nature said so. Then we went out for a ride, and I felt much better. My son Alan was married and had two beautiful children, Mark and Kara, so I understood that I was crying for nothing. Two months later I went to Brazil, and my cousin told me about a lady doctor who practiced natural medicine. I told her that I was feeling ugly, depressed, and sad. I told her that I hated the word 'sex' and I felt alone.

She said: "You not the first, nor the last, woman with these symptoms. At least you don't have hot flashes, than you really would feel worse."

Long story short, she gave me some drops from herbs. After one week, I was feeling better. It was like a miracle. I took those drops for a year, and then I stopped. I never had hot flashes, never gained weight, and my skin was beautiful.

But I started early. If you decide to take natural medicine, you have to understand that it takes a little longer for you to be your old self again, but it is safe. Not only that: your body will still be the same, with no extra fat. Lots of women take anti-depression pills and hormones, and the results are the worst. So try natural medicine for menopause. It works for everyone. There is no risk, and you will feel great.

Menopause is woman's worst enemy, so take your enemy out of your life. Be happy, and feel beautiful again. Remember that you are getting better each day, but you must love yourself every day as well. Exercise, take calcium, go to the doctor for regular checkups, and look at the mirror every morning and tell yourself how healthy, happy, beautiful and blessed you are. Say that looking straight into your eyes. Believe me, it works!

Words have tremendous power, so say positive words, so that positive things will happen. When negative thoughts come just sing and start to think beautiful things.

Instead of being jealous of a friend that looks great, be happy and make yourself look better in a nice way. Today things are so easy for us, so we can correct the lines on our face and eyes. Today is affordable to everyone, but please don't blow up your lips. There are other ways to pick them up. As far as your body fat is concerned, stay away from dairy as much as you can. That will eliminate that fat around your tummy. I will give a health diet at the end.

Most importantly, from 50 till 60, you will go through so many little things. Don't let them bother you, because one day we said those same words that we are going to hear now: it's part of life.

Things that will bother you, which you are just going to let go:

Two friends talking: "This guy had the nerve to ask me out! He was 36! I said to myself he is too old, who does he think he is?" Her friend said, "I guess they don't have a mirror in their house."

1. When you go to a department store, and a girl ask you: "Ma'am, can I help you find something?"

2. You go have your makeup done with a girl that has no business working in the industry, and after talking to you for a while, she says, "You are just like my mom."

3. "When you were young did you use lots of makeup? You have such beautiful skin. I hope when I get to be your age, my skin will look like yours."

I've heard many of these comments at the counter where I worked, and I used to tell the girls: "We do not talk about age to clients. And besides, you might be 25, but you look 30 with all that junk on your face."

As you can see, after a certain age we start to take things personally. I used to too, until I realized what I was doing. I was hurting myself! As I told you in the beginning of the book, we are our worst enemies.

If you are divorced, or never married, I want you to know, and I assure you, that there is someone for you out there. Just don't be too picky, and never say that you don't want to be married, because nobody wants to be alone. Again, words have power, and our tendency after 50 is to find something wrong with everybody we meet. In our beautiful age, love is a mix of friendship, companionship, and affection. When someone is there for us, our values change. That's true love.

When people tell me that I don't look my age, because Brazilian women are different, that's not true. I love myself, and I feel beautiful, young, and easygoing with men. I like to dance, and I am happy most the time. I have also lived in the United States for 42 years. I always say that of course a tropical climate has a lot to do with people's attitudes, but for me, I try to find beauty in everything. That means I am in love and happy with myself. I know my other half is on the way, and I say thank you God for the wonderful husband you chose for my life, even though I don't have him yet. Don't be like those other women that say, "Men are no good. They are all the same. All they want are young girls!" This is not true. Don't hang up on bars. Go once a week to a nice restaurant where there are beautiful people. And if you can't spend the money, share a plate with your girlfriend. If you want to meet a nice man, go to a nice place. Dress sexy but not vulgar. What is yours will come to you.

Now, let's talk about beauty! Hair should be a little below the shoulders. Volume makes you look younger. Don't be afraid to change your looks - change is good. If you have a large forehead, bangs will be great. Don't forget your eyebrows: they should not be thin. If they don't grow, use a pencil and then eyebrow powder to make it look natural. Smoky eyes are okay, but go easy. Use light foundation, bronzer, and a little blush. Lips should not be too dark, and not too light.

And you know what? Be yourself, and just make sure to never to let the person you are interested in feel that you need someone. That's the first step to chase him away. Learn to listen, and watch the words that come out of your mouth.

I want to wish all the women from 50 to 55 all the best. I wish I knew all of you, to be able to guide you when you feel blue, but keep this book with you at all times, and at the end, I will give you my e-mail for emergencies. Okay?

I love you all very much!

Xoxoxoxoxoxoxoxoxoxoxoxoxoxoxo!

XO

Chapter Eight

AGE 55 TO 65

Between the ages of 55 to 65, you go through big changes. Personally I think this is very difficult for most women, but if you just try to understand that you are maturing instead of getting older, life will be much easier for you. I know many women that at the age of 65 look like they're 50 instead. You know why? They don't worry about the numbers like most women do. Sure, it is easy to say, right? Wrong, you are as young or as old as you feel. I know that you go through so many changes, that at times you feel depressed. I will give you some examples.

You look in the mirror, and find that your face has changed. Your neck and lines on your face can be corrected. Today there are many ways for you to look younger, without looking artificial, but the most important thing is your mind. Are you going to feel sorry for yourself every time you see a young girl pass by with a perfect figure, wearing a miniskirt that makes men turn around, and everything in place, saying to yourself: "They don't look at me like that!"

So, we had our days, now men look at us with different eyes: a mature look. Every day I meet women in their fifties and early sixties, looking great and beautiful.

There's a gym for everyone. So kick depression, and love yourself.

Let's go back to our time of glory, and feel good about it? Ok! 70's hot pants with boots, and a long colt. It was winter - how great we looked with our popcorn blouses, gaucho pants, and knickers. Remember the velvet knickers with a turtleneck sweater? What about Macy's? Back then it was a fantastic store! B'altmans, and Bloomingdale's - on Saturdays it was the place to be to meet a guy, and right across the street there was Yellow Fingers for the afternoon. What about P.J. Clarks, with their great hamburgers, surrounded by famous writers, and gorgeous looking men? Back than they would by our lunch, then dinner at night.

Remember the Greek nightclubs Adonis and Dionysius? They would send a rose to the table when they liked a girl, and we dance and break plates. Blue Angel was a great nightclub with a live show. Those were great times: people would fall in love and get married in those days.

Commonwealth was another Sunday nightclub to meet the guys. We looked beautiful and didn't have to show our breasts. Implants were rare back then. And for good eating? We had Kenny's steak pub; Palm, Pen and Pencil; the Four Seasons restaurant; Peter Lugers in Williamsburg; Nanni, for the best Italian food; Il Valletto; Amalfi, another great Italian restaurant; and Brasserrie was open 24 hours.

For holidays, Miami Beach Fontainblue hotel was the best hotel in Miami. It had a great night club, and New Yorkers would go there for holidays. There was the Forge steak house, and if you liked to dance the RealCuban salsa, it was the best.

Moving on to the eighties: Studio 54 and Barry Manilow, with his romantic songs. Those were days that will never come back, but they were the good old days. Most of my friends from that time are still beautiful.

What I am trying to say is that we had our time. For our generation it was the best: we were romantic, soft, and, most of all, happy.

Now it is time for the new generation. Our children grew. Some got married, and we are beautiful grandmas looking good. So instead of wanting to be in your twenties again, enjoy who you are now. Believe me, we are still getting better. Each day we mature more and more, so just be in shape, go the gym, do yoga (which is great for the mind). Love yourself every single day, even when you feeling blue. We are winners! We survived the most difficult years, and here we are.

Some of you that didn't get married don't feel bad. What is yours is reserved for you. Who said there's a right age to find a partner? That's a no-no. I see some of my friends meeting their other half now. Some want to get married, or live together, or stay independent. You make the choice. The truth is that nobody wants to be alone. I don't blame them: real love is friendship and companionship. Sex is not so important anymore. We want affection, to hold hands and be there for each other. Of course, going out dancing, watching movies, and traveling is fun. Don't stay home thinking: "Now I am old." Most sickness comes from the mind. A healthy mind is a healthy body.

If you are over weight, lose it. Make yourself beautiful. I can make a 65-year-old look 50, and so on. You know why? Because I know what its good for you, especially after I get to know you for a few minutes.

Don't ever put yourself down. You are winners, not losers. I know some people are more successful than you. Maybe you didn't fight for what you wanted. So do it now! At the age of 62, George Washington became the first President of the United States, and he had a very sad life before he accomplished that.

So why not you? You can be anything you want. Just focus.

Now, makeup: foundation, and a little bronzing powder and blush, will always give you a youthful look. Light eye shadow all over - not white, but bone color, with no shimmer at all. On the outside corner of your eyes, a darker color to bring up the eyes. Soft eyeliner, mascara, medium color lips, not shimmer, full eyebrows. If you do not have much hair, again I will say use a pencil that matches your hair color, followed by eyebrow powder. Hair shoulder length, no dark color. Soft highlights will look great. Dress with common sense, exercise, keep your mind busy with creative things, and you will see great results. Dancing is good for you, and music is a must. Always avoid talking about sickness with people. The word has power! And don't forget the mirror exercise every morning. Look into the mirror, into inside your eyes, and say the magic words: Laura, you are beautiful and I love you. Today is the best day of my life. I love and approve of myself just as I am. But remember, never get out of bed before thanking God for health and one more day, and thank Him for being in your life every single day. He is and always be your best friend, the one that loves you eternally. Okay, but why is my friend is sick, while mean people are not? Don't worry about other people. There are mysteries in this life that don't belong to us.

Live your life to the fullest. From 70 to 80 we are going to still be beautiful. Remember: healthy mind, healthy body.

Xoxoxoxoxoxoxoxoxoxoxo!

Chapter Nine

MATURE WOMEN

When I wrote about mature women, I though about myself, and all women in their thirties, forties, fifties or sixties. I also wrote about the 20 year olds, they're so beautiful, youthful and innocent, but smart in their own way. They are just so loveable, especially when they ask you for advice. That's when we are able to share our experiences with them. I wish I could spend time helping these beauties whenever they need me.

Now, I wrote something beautiful about mature women. I hope you enjoy it:

Mature women doesn't provoke
She's provocative

Mature women doesn't anticipate
Waits for the right moment
Mature women doesn't think quantity

She prefers quality
Mature women is not intelligent

She is more than that, she is wise
Mature women will never judge
She will look around and analyze

Mature women never guess
She has great deal of perception

Mature women doesn't make sex
She is a master in the art of lovemaking

Mature women is not easy
She is very flexible

Anyway, most mature women have a combination of all possible beauties.

I hope you were able to appreciate the beautiful words I wrote for you.

Xoxoxoxoxoxoxoxoxoxoxoxoxoxoxoxoxoxoxoxo

How to take care of your skin

Oily skin

It doesn't matter how old you are. You have to take care of your skin the proper way, so you won't take away the natural oil of your skin.

At night remove your make up with oil-free makeup remover. Make sure your remover also removes eye makeup.

After your makeup is totally off, apply your lotion, always using a cotton pad. After the lotion, wash your face with a neutral soap; it can be liquid or bar soap. Most important is very cold water: not only to keep your skin firm, but to keep your pores closed. When your pores start to open, you have to be careful with acne, which is enemy number one of oily skin.

Once the skin is totally clean, put your eye cream on with no moisturizer. This is so your pores are able to breath.

Morning: eye cream and oil-free moisturizer with SPF. Then apply your makeup. Very important: I recommend loose powder. If you do like to use powder, pressed powder for oily skin is a no-no that clogs the pores. But if you insist, make sure you do not use a powder puff. Use a fluffy powder brush very softly all over your face. Just enough to take the shine away.

If you do use foundation, make sure you use an oil-free primer. This prevents the foundation from getting inside your pores.

Doing your home facial

I recommend that you have a professional facial three times a year. You don't have to buy all the items she is going to recommend. Just get a regular facial. If you have a serious skin problem, the best thing is a good dermatologist.

Now let's go back to your own home facial. This should be done once a week.

Usually, I recommend a home facial when you have time to relax.

After your skin is totally clean, with a wet face, apply a mild face scrub very gently all over the face. Always avoid the eye area. You can find face scrub in department stores, or in a drugstore. There are good ones on drugstores, and they are very inexpensive. Just make sure the one you purchase is mild.

After you are done, use a cotton pad with warm water to remove all the scrub from your face. Right after, wash your face with very cold water until you feel that its totally clean. The cold water will always keep your skin firm and pores closed.

Now, I am going to teach you how to make a mask. You should do this every week with your home facial.

1. A full-size teaspoon of organic shredded oatmeal

2. A full-size teaspoon of organic honey

3. A full-size teaspoon of sour cream

Mix everything well. Put it all over your face with a brush. Don't use your fingers, and avoid the eye area under the lower eye lashes. Lay down for 45 minutes. No talking and no walking: just relax, and think about beautiful things.

After 45 minutes, use a cotton pad with warm water to remove the mask. Right after, wash with cold water, until the skin is totally clean. You will feel great! This mask is excellent. The oatmeal rejuvenates the skin cells, the honey firms the skin, and the sour cream helps to soften the honey.

I've learned all this from a friend of mine, one of the best dermatologists in Brazil. Every time I see him, I learn something new. So I hope you will do your own home facial every week. You will see the difference!

Xoxoxoxoxoxoxoxoxoxoxoxoxoxoxoxoxo!

Normal to dry skin

20 to 65 years

Normal skin should be treated as normal from the age of 18 until the age of 25. After that, you should take care of your skin as if were normal to dry. Years ago, we ate properly, the weather was different, girls didn't drink and smoke like today, and they didn't use heavy makeup. The sun on your face is pure poison, and stress plays with your hormones. So for all these reasons and more, starting 25, is normal to dry.

At night time, remove your makeup with a three-in-one makeup remover, for the face, eyes, and moisturizer. If you can't buy this a department store, you can get a good one at a well-known drugstore.

Massage your face (go easy on the eyes), and remove with a cotton pad soaked in warm water. Use your lotion, and, at last, wash your face with a neutral soap bar or liquid, and wash off with loads of cold water. This will keep your skin firm and pores closed.

Put your eye cream on, and then it's bed time.

I know that some people don't agree with me when I say no face moisturizer when you go to sleep. I will explain why.

During the day you use face moisturizer with SPF, eye cream, and makeup. You go to work, and by the time you get home you are totally stressed out inside. Your skin also suffers. The only time you are relaxed is when you sleeping. Your body is calm, and your pores, are able to breath. I never used moisturizer at night and I have a fantastic skin. When you wake up, you will feel your skin fresh and healthy. If you feel the need for a night moisturizer, just do it, as long as it is SPF-free.

In the morning, use moisturizer with SPF, eye cream, and face primer before foundation, tinted moisturizer, or everything else you use. Have a great day!

Doing your home facial

I recommend a professional facial three times a year, and, once again, you don't have to buy everything that is recommended to you. After you have a facial done by a professional, they will always tell you that you need to buy almost everything. This is wrong! Don't do it unless you really want it. The best thing to do if you think something is wrong with your skin is to go to a dermatologist.

1. After your skin is totally clean, you should wet your face a little and apply your face scrub or gomage all over the face. Always avoid the eye area.

2. With a warm cotton pad, remove all the scrub or gomage. Right after, wash your face with very cold water.

Now you can use any mask that you think is good for your skin type. I am going to give you 2 mask recipes that are fantastic, and will give you new skin that you will notice right away.

Oatmeal Mask

1. One teaspoon full of organic grain oatmeal.

2. One teaspoon full of organic honey.

3. One teaspoon full of sour cream.

Mix everything in a cup and put all over your face with a brush. Always avoid the eye area. Lie down for 40 minutes and just relax. After that, wash your face with warm water, and right after, cold water. Eye cream and that's all.

Egg Mask

(Not for oily skin)

1. One egg yolk.

2. One teaspoon full of organic honey.

3. One teaspoon full of fresh squeezed lemon juice.

The egg and the honey firm the skin, and the lemon softens the yolk and the honey.

Enjoy it!

Exercises

As I told you earlier, I am going to give you some exercises that will help day by day.

As you know, in order to love someone, you must love yourself first. Sometimes we make the mistake of being with someone we don't love, for the simple reason of not being alone. Is this true or false?

I can tell stories that I know of about women who don't love themselves. But that is not the case. My concern is to help you find yourself, in order to have a good quality of life.

When you wake up, before you get out of bed, make sure you say thank you to God for your life, and your health.

After that just do what you usually do: yoga, meditation, what ever.

Now, as I mentioned in the beginning of the book, we are both our best friends, and our worst enemies. When you are happy, you are nice to everyone, you feel like you in heaven, and everything is perfect.

When you are upset, your face changes, you are rude to people, and with these attitudes, you bring your enemy (your own self) into your life. That's when we say things that we will regret later on, break up relationships, eat, go into depression, think the whole world is against us, and develop inferiority complexes. We become negative, and do all sorts of bad things. Without knowing, you will bring all of these things into reality. You speak those famous words, "life is not fair," and then you start asking Why? Why? Why? But life is beautiful, and we make our life the way we want.

Sometimes we don't have the right person next to us to help us when we need them, but who is better than your own self to make things work the way you want? You are your best friend. You must chase your enemy away every time something happens that makes you upset. Is it easy? Yes, it is very easy. I have seen many girls get away from their own enemy. This is very serious: you can help yourself and be in total control of your emotions, in order to have a fantastic life.

The Mirror

After you wash your face and brush your teeth, look in the mirror. What do you see? The beautiful you.

Look straight into your eyes and tell yourself everything you want for your life. Bring everything into your life, as if they are already happening. For example:

I love myself, I have total control of my emotions, and today I am having a great day. I am losing all my extra pounds with my new diet (if you are overweight).

Go on with your affirmations, always looking into your eyes, and smile. It works! I did it and I had great success. Just believe in yourself, even when your day is not going as well as you expected. Tell yourself: all is well. I am very happy! Bring into your life words that you want to become real. Our minds are powerful. Just make sure you will use good thoughts only, and I assure you, you will always be a winner.

Do this everyday, even when you feel blue. Don't give up on you. You will see miracles, I promise.

All About Me

I was born in Sao Paulo, Brazil, but I came to New York when I was 17 years old. I love Brazil, but the most important years of my life were spent here. When I go to Brazil every year on vacation, my cousin always asks me if I like New York more than I like Brazil. I always give her the same answer.

"I spent most of my life in New York, so i have to say that my home is here. But I love Brazil, and everything about it. I am proud to be born there. I miss you all, but my life is in New York."

My mother went to be with the Lord when I was 16 years old. One year later, my father followed her. I loved them both very much. They were the best, but until this day, I think of my father almost every day, and I still I cry. He was very special. Unfortunately, we only agree with them once they are gone.

For those of you who are lucky to have good parents, be good, and spend time loving them. Because once they are gone, they are gone forever.

I didn't come from a religious family. My father said that men created religion, but there was only one God, and he loves us all the way we are. Before I went to sleep, my mother made sure I said my prayers. The funny part was that I thought that Jesus was a little boy and God was the big father. My father told me that on the day I die, don't be afraid, because God is my Eternal Father. He will always take care of me.

Every time he said that I cried, because I thought he was trying to tell me that he was going to die. But he always made sure to tell me that it was just an explanation.

As a child, I always liked to daydream. I was good in everything I did, except in school. I never liked to study, but I was ok. I was very popular, especially when there were events. They always chose me because I was so adorable, and full of life. My dream as a child was to be a movie actress, just to be close to my favorite actor Alain Delon. He was the love of my life. I collected all of his pictures. He had the most beautiful face I have ever seen on a man. I remember I was 14 years old when he got married to Natalie Delon. I cried so much.

My father said, "My princess, he doesn't even know that you exist. One day you are going to meet a nice boy, so don't cry."

Long story short, I didn't go to school for two days. My school friends came to visit me, because they knew how much I loved him. After that, I threw away all of his pictures, and never talked about him again. But until this day, I have to say that he has the most beautiful face I have ever seen.

Back than you had to be 18 in order to see pictures with love scenes. Some of my favorite actresses were Ursula Andress, Eizabeth Taylor, Claudia Cardinale, and Sofia Loren. These were the most beautiful.

I was very creative. I learned how to sew in school. I made beautiful dresses for myself, but I could never make a pattern. I would cut straight from the fabric. But they came out beautiful; all my friends went crazy with my dresses, because I created my own styles. I was a beautiful girl, if I may say so. I was always tanned, I had beautiful long hair, and my hair was dark brown. Brown, with gold highlights, all from the sun. When I went in the sun I used to put lemon in my hair, so it would get all these different colors.

Aside from all that, I always lived in my own world. I would talk to myself in front of the mirror saying everything I wanted, such as: "You are beautiful; you are the best in everything you do." I would go on and on. My father saw me one day and said: "You are right, keep on doing that."

Imagine I was 15 years old, and I really loved everything about me. Some of my friends would tell me that my sign was Leo, that's why I thought I was the best. This is wrong. I thought it was the best for me, not better than everybody else.

That's when I started to understand that there was jealousy, and that is no good. When you waste your time being jealous of people, you will never grow in life. One thing is to admire somebody, but jealousy doesn't take you any where. When I was with my friends, I would observe them and I was able to see what kind of a person they were. That way, I would eliminate them as a friend. Of course I did this in a nice way. I had the gift of being able to talk to people and look in their eyes, and know if the person was sincere or not. Don't ask me how, but I was always right. I knew a lot of girls, but only had one real friend. We were like sisters, always together.

I was very popular with the boys, but I was also very smart. I used to see the girls run after them, and they would lose interest, so I always did the opposite. When I liked a boy, I would give a fast look and keep on walking, and they were always after me. The girls used to ask me why they liked me if I didn't even talk to them. I would tell them that boys don't like when girls are all over them. But they didn't care, and they were always crying. Not me - I loved myself so much, and I knew that I would know who the right boy for me was.

I always had a head on my shoulders. Something always bothered me, though: I would go to weddings with my parents, and the couples were always so in love. But after the girl had a baby, the husband was already looking at other women. Then I realized that the wife got fat and all she did was talk about the baby. It's fine, but if I was her, I would look beautiful for husband and myself, so he wouldn't have to look at other women. I was very critical, and I already knew in my mind how I would behave after I was married.

I am talking about 40 years ago. Imagine now how things are! But I still think the same way. The ball game starts after you get married, before it's all roses. I knew many husbands that had other women on the side, and that made me grow smart, and follow my father's famous words: "Never go to sleep angry with your husband, and never let him go to work in the morning upset."

I always enjoyed spending time by myself. I was happy having a good relationship with myself. It helped me understand people, and have a world that was mine. I was able to see ugly things, and people, without judgment. I believe that people have the right to choose their way of life, if you choose wrong, life itself will show you sooner or later. I always had God as my best friend. When I was sad I ran to him, and also when I was happy. I think that's one of the reasons that I was always able to forgive people that hurt me.

I always say treat people the way you like to be treated. I am far from being perfect, but I love people, I love to see everyone happy, and that makes my life go smooth.

My dream, since a young age, was to make every woman look beautiful. I am able to transform a person in such a way that sometimes I surprise myself. And the inside part is that I can always give good advice, when I am asked to do so.

I was married twice. I have two beautiful sons, Alan, who is 40 years old, and Joshua, who is

35 years old. When people see us together, they don't believe we are mother and sons. I look very young, and I say that in a good way. I believe in healthy mind, healthy body, and healthy soul. Therefore, I will look young for a long time.

I also have four grandchildren from my son Alan: Mark, 19 and Kara, 16 from Alan, and Isaac, 9, and Esther, 6, from Joshua. The way things are going, I will probably be a young great-grandmother.

I will be 59 years old on August 6. I am a Leo woman. If you believe in signs, you know that Leos are usually very good and sincere friends.

I have been divorced for a few years. I divorced my husbands; not because they had other women, but for reasons that I would rather keep to myself. My second husband, Joshua's father, was the love of my life. We loved each other so very much. He is no longer in this world, but we were good friends after our divorce, and I will always remember him as if he was alive.

Now I am ready to meet Mr. Right. I will continue with my books, and I will try to make all women of this world understand that they are all winners, and that they are not getting older, but getting better and better everyday.

I would like to say that I wrote this book with love and care for every woman, and I hope you enjoyed this time we've spent together.

www.ingramcontent.com/pod-product-compliance
Lightning Source LLC
Chambersburg PA
CBHW020350290526
45785CB00005B/2207